Chakras for Beginners

How to Balance Chakras, Strengthen Aura, and Radiate Energy

Victoria Lane

©2014

Your Free Gift!

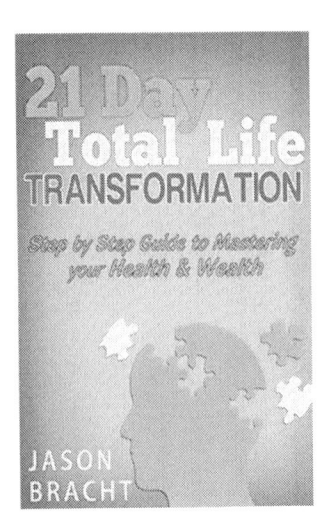

Our publishing team has collaborated on an E-Book that I believe will help anyone who wants to make a lasting change in their life. The title is *21 Day Total Life Transformation*. All you have to do is go to JasonBracht.com enter your email address and I will deliver it directly to your inbox.

This resource will help you get the most out of life – It lays out step by step techniques that can help dig you out of any rut.

To get instant access to these incredible tools and resources, click the link below:

Click here for the FREE 21 Day Total Life Transformation Book

Table of Contents

The energy inside your body

    What is an aura?

    What are chakras?

Understanding the seven main chakras

    The first chakra or the root chakra

    The second chakra or the sacral chakra

    The third chakra or the solar plexus chakra

    The fourth chakra or the heart chakra

    The fifth chakra or the throat chakra

    The sixth chakra or the brow chakra

    The seventh chakra or the crown chakra

Balancing the seven chakras

    Chakra mudras

    Using the Mudras

    Chakra chants

    Bija Mantras or the seed mantras

Yoga for chakras

The final word

The energy inside your body

Each and every living being is infused with a universal energy that nourishes and connects life. This energy has traditionally been called by various names, such as mana, prana and chi. Human beings are surrounded by an *'invisible energy field'* that is comprised of this energy.

Did you know that the manner in which your mind functions and you express your emotions, your spiritual life, and the operating system of your physical body – necessarily, each and every life process in your body, mind and soul is supported via this energy field?

The energy in this energy field is active, intelligent and full of life. It is this conscious energy that appears as an indicator of your universal consciousness which is also the source of this entire universe. This energy, just like everything else in the universe, originates from the *field of pure consciousness,* which is also the spiritual origin of life. Infinite love, unlimited consciousness, infinite health, power, wellness and knowledge are born from this *field of pure consciousness*.

Each one of us possesses this consciousness individually and yet, each one of us is connected and ultimately one.

Your association to this greatest spiritual reality lies within you; it lies in your vital nature which tells you that you are pure consciousness, with unlimited power and knowledge inside your body.

This energy field is made up of the *aura* (which manifests itself in seven layers) and the *chakra system* (which comprises of the seven major chakras). It acts as a seven step connection or the bridge between life and the field of pure consciousness present in this world. This energy field brings to life the unlimited potential and the infinite power which is a characteristic of our spiritual being. It indicates and regulates the manner in which the life force or 'chi' or 'prana' exists within your field of pure consciousness and manifests itself in your worldly life.

You have the capability to demonstrate great health at each level – mental, physical, emotional and spiritual – only if this energy field stays healthy, clear and free from all defects.

The intrinsic harmony and health of your mind, body and soul, the awareness of your spiritual self and your highest potential manifests in your life by virtue of a quorate connection to this field of pure consciousness which enables the flow of these traits. A number of times, however, certain *energetic defects* appear in this energy field. An impure, weak, impaired, blocked or unbalanced flow of energy prevents your connection with the ultimate spiritual reality or your field of pure consciousness. This field of pure consciousness is actually your true self.

The cause of these energetic defects can be traced to a psychological or a physical trauma. Any traumatic experience or a damaging life incidence or an unhealthy relationship in your past (this also includes your past life) may sometimes not get completely assimilated by your psyche. This may result in excitation of an energy field with energetic defects. These energetic defects may disable you from establishing a complete connection between your true self and the ultimate reality, leaving some severe biases, which may also mean some unpleasant changes in your personality.

They also establish unhealthy energies within your aura and chakras. As a result of this, the strong and healthy energy which is originally present in your energy field becomes compromised. This results in three kinds of defects:

- Severe trauma to personality which may also include some suppressed memories
- Basic energetic defects within your aura and chakra system which may include negative emotions and thoughts
- Attack by unhealthy and impure energy which is sometimes self-generated and sometimes enforced by others

Therefore, it can be said that these three defects very often exist together and are closely inter related.

They also prevent the complete and healthy expression of your self-potential and eliminate the natural environment of energetic health which is a basic requirement for emotional, mental, physical and spiritual well-being.

What is an aura?

Did you know that everything in this universe is just a vibration? Every atom, part of an atom, electron, proton and neutron is a vibration. In fact, your thoughts and consciousness are also vibrations. You can, therefore, term the Aura as *'an electro-photonic vibration response of an object to some external excitation (such as an ambient light for example)'*. It may also be called an energy field that engulfs, penetrates and spreads out beyond your physical body. It is electromagnetic (electric and magnetic) and comprises of various types of live and intelligent frequencies or vibrations. This electromagnetic radiation spans from microwave, infrared (IR) to UV light. The low frequency microwave and infrared part of the spectrum (body heat) is related to the levels of physical functioning of your body (DNA structure, metabolism, circulation etc.) whereas the high frequency or the UV part is connected to your conscious activity such as creativity, sense of humor, intentions, thinking and emotions.

An aura not only surrounds every living thing including plants, animals and humans, it also engulfs each inanimate object including the objects created by man, and the earth, moon, sun, stars and all planets in this universe. The human aura has layers of emotional, mental, physical and spiritual elements. The aura around conscious or living beings may vary with time, and at other times it may change very quickly. However, the aura around non-living beings remains fixed and may be altered by your conscious intent.

Auras are made up of all the primary colors of the rainbow at any given time and may change their color depending upon the emotions that you are experiencing. Your aura is therefore made up of various shades of colors that keep changing constantly. This demonstrates constant alterations in your emotions and thoughts.

Loving and happy thoughts enhance your aura whereas angry and sad thoughts diminish it. The size of the aura adjusts itself based on the density of the population where you live.

The most important thing about an aura is the fact that it contains almost every bit of information about an object. The intensity and color of the aura, especially above and surrounding your head has a definite meaning. Mastering the skill of watching someone's aura can enable you to experience the person's thoughts before he or she expresses them verbally. You can spot a lie almost always because aura cannot be faked.

It also becomes your spiritual signature. An individual with a clean and bright aura demonstrates a spiritually advanced personality. He may not even be aware of this! An individual with a dark or gray aura demonstrates unclear intentions.

What are chakras?

Chakras can be termed as the spinning wheels of electric energy in your body. These wheels are made up of various colors and are responsible for a number of functions that connect your body to your energy field and the broader cosmic energy field.

The chakras are linking mechanisms between the meridian system and the auric field inside your physical body. They also serve as a connection between the different levels of auras and the cosmic energy field. They impact the flow of energy into your physical body. Chakras are termed as 'energy transformers' because they can absorb the primary energy from the atmosphere and transport it into your body via the energy channels. This vitalizes your physical body along with nurturing a feeling of self-consciousness within your spiritual being.

The ancient prophets mentioned the chakra system as a pillar of energy centers that extends from the base of your spine to the top of your head. Your body contains seven major chakras or energy centers. It also has one hundred and twenty two minor chakras. The location of each chakra is related to a portion of your body's anatomy. It is also connected to a specific color.

The seven major chakras are

- The Root Chakra - located at the base of the spine
- The Sacral Chakra - located at the navel

- The Solar Plexus Chakra- located in your solar plexus
- The Heart Chakra- located within your heart
- The Throat Chakra- located within your throat
- The Brow or Third Eye Chakra- located at the center of your forehead and
- The Crown Chakra- located at the top of your head

These are linked to each other.

When either one of these main chakras goes out of balance, implying it gets under-worked or over-worked, it leads to a physical, emotional or mental impact on your body. It may even impact one of the neighboring chakras. This imbalance is caused by the negativity and the impurities present in your external or internal environment and their aura. Since your chakras are dependent and related to each other for balance and harmony, it becomes imperative to understand the various aspects of these seven chakras and then work on them.

Understanding the seven main chakras

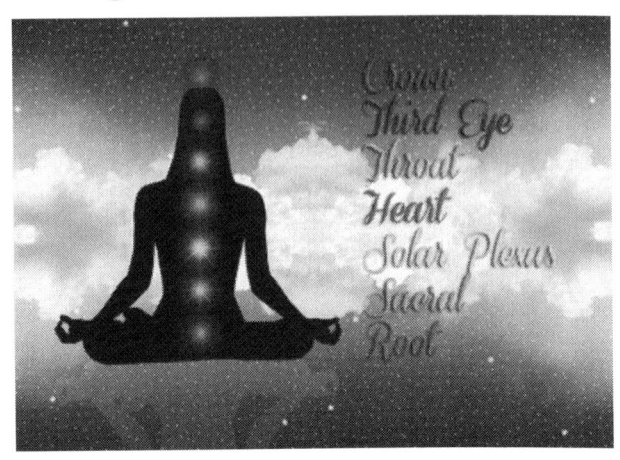

Chakras are related to functions your body performs and are influenced by specific circumstances in your life. The manner in which you handle various life circumstances is also influenced through your chakras. As a vital life force, the chakras are sites through which you absorb, distribute and receive life energy. Chakras may become deficient or excessive through certain internal habits or external life situations.

These imbalances may be temporary or chronic. A chronic imbalance may be a result of past experiences, pain, stress, childhood memories or cultural mindset. An example here can be a child whose family moves location every two years. This child may not understand how one can feel grounded in one location and this may result in a deficient first chakra, which will neither receive the adequate amount of energy nor will be able to spread its own energy. This creates a sense of emotional and physical imbalance.

An over balanced or excessive chakra impacts your ability to operate in a healthy manner and can become a major dominating force in your life. A great example to understand this is your fifth chakra or the throat chakra. An over-balanced fifth chakra or the throat chakra may lead to an extremely talkative child and an under balanced fifth chakra may lead to a child who experiences difficulty in communication.

Before we get into the basics of chakra healing, let us understand each chakra in detail:

The first chakra or the root chakra

Sanskrit name	Muladhara
Where is it located?	It is located towards the base of your spine and in the region of your pubic bone. It faces downwards towards your feet
Which organs does this chakra govern?	Reproductive organs, spinal cord, immune system, adrenal gland, rectum, legs and feet
How does it influence your body, mind and soul?	Mental stability, sense of security, sensuality, sexuality
How does an imbalance of this chakra impact you?	An imbalance may result in varicose veins, lower back pain, depression, immunity related disorders, rectal tumors, low self-esteem and security issues
Symbol	Square

The Muladhara or the root chakra ensures that you are linked to this earth and serves as the very base of your existence. The feeling of being rooted at one place or being grounded is a result of a balanced first chakra. It serves as a foundation for your emotional health, mental strength and physical vitality. Your passion in life, great physical endurance and an amazing mental balance are a result of a clear first energy center. You should listen to your root chakra if you are faced in an important decision making scenario. An uncomfortable feeling sends you a message to be attentive and re-evaluate your decision whereas a pleasant feeling indicates that your decision can enhance your safety along with nourishing your body and soul.

This chakra is stimulated and energized by the color 'RED'. Red gemstones such as ruby and garnet along with red clothing can provide the much required red energy boost to your root chakra. Red foods and drinks such as radish, beetroot, onion, red pepper, red beans and spices such as paprika can provide you a grounded impact through your root chakra. Certain aromatherapy oils such as juniper or sandalwood can also trigger this energy center.

The second chakra or the sacral chakra

Sanskrit name	Swadhisthana or Svadisthana
Where is it located?	It is located in the sacrum, below your navel and in your lower abdomen

Which organs does this chakra govern?	Sexual organs, gonad gland, liver, stomach, gall bladder, kidney, upper intestine, adrenal glands, spleen and middle spine
How does it influence your body, mind and soul?	Joyfulness, enthusiasm, reproduction and creativity
How does an imbalance of this chakra impact you?	An imbalance may result in anger, apathy, hatred, menace, greed, guilt, control, power, immorality, pelvic pain, gynaecological problems, urinary problems and libido issues
Symbol	Up-turned crescent

The second chakra or the Swadhisthana is your creativity, finances, personal power and sexuality center. This energy center connects you to your inner child, your feelings and sensualities. It is tied to physical feelings of passion, love and sexuality. This chakra also facilitates the act of giving and receiving.

A healthy second chakra empowers you to tap into your source of creative energy that enables you to compose beautiful music, nurture an innovative business proposal or create a secure and loving family life. An imbalance in this chakra results in a blockage in your creative powers, which creates a sense of emptiness or dryness.

The key color of this chakra is 'ORANGE' and this enables it to enhance its powers. You can arouse the energy of this chakra through deep tissue massages, trying a variety of food flavors or embracing sentiments arising through viewing of emotional movies.

This chakra is stimulated and energized by the color 'ORANGE'. Wearing orange colored clothes and gemstones such as coral or carnelian elevates the power of this chakra. Foods that are orange in color such as oranges, mangoes, cinnamon and passion fruit can nourish your creative and sensual center. Aromatherapy oils such as mandarin, orange, melissa and mandarin can also boost the powers of your sacral chakra.

The third chakra or the solar plexus chakra

Sanskrit name	Manipura
Where is it located?	It is located in your stomach area just above the navel

Which organs does this chakra govern?	Upper abdomen, liver, pancreas, middle spine, gall bladder, adrenals, kidney, spleen, stomach, small intestine
How does it influence your body, mind and soul?	Self-confidence, growth, self-control, humor, self-power, ego power and digestion
How does an imbalance of this chakra impact you?	An imbalance may result in diabetes, constipation, digestive problems, ulcers, self-esteem, oversensitivity to criticism, self-image fears, nervousness and poor memory
Symbol	Descending triangle

The third chakra or the solar plexus chakra defines your self-esteem. Your mental awareness, ego, optimism, will-power and confidence originate from your solar plexus chakra. The solar plexus energy center also rules your concentration power and your ability to comprehend things. Your instincts originate from the solar plexus chakra. A free flow of energy through this chakra brings in the confidence to fulfill your desires and intentions. A blockage in this energy center, however, results in rendering you frustrated and powerless.

This chakra is stimulated and energized by the color 'YELLOW'. Wearing yellow colored clothes, gold and gemstones such as topaz and amber facilitate the release of healing vibrations from this energy center. Grains such as rice, sunflower seeds and flax seeds along with dairy products such as cheese, milk and yogurt and spices such as turmeric, ginger, fennel, cumin, and chamomile arouse this chakra. . Aromatherapy oils such as lemon, rosemary, grapefruit and bergamot can also boost the powers of your sacral chakra.

The fourth chakra or the heart chakra

Sanskrit name	Anahata
Where is it located?	It is located near the center of your chest
Which organs does this chakra govern?	Lungs, blood, circulatory system, thymus, diaphragm, heart, oesophagus, shoulders, arms, legs and breast
How does it influence your body, mind and soul?	Compassion, forgiveness, passion, devotion, love for self, love for others, circulatory system

How does an imbalance of this chakra impact you?	Lung cancer, pneumonia, breast cancer, shoulder problems, confidence issues, envy, fear, hate, despair, confidence, passivity and jealously
Symbol	Intertwined descending and ascending triangles

The fourth chakra or the heart chakra is a storehouse of your energy system and the center of healing and love. This energy center is connected to your emotions and empowers you to give and love unconditionally. It also facilitates any emotional healing that is required and serves as a connection between your body and soul. You feel connected to everyone in our life when your fourth chakra is open and flowing. However, an obstruction may lead to a sense of alienation and loneliness.

This chakra is associated with the color 'GREEN' and sometimes 'PINK'. Green colored clothes and gemstones such as emerald, peridot and jade elevate the positive effects of this heart chakra. Foods and drinks such as broccoli, spinach, squash and green tea and herbs such as thyme, basil, cilantro and parsley can awaken the powers of your heart chakra. Aromatherapy oils such as eucalyptus, tea tree, pine, spearmint and cedar wood can also stimulate the powers of your heart chakra.

The fifth chakra or the throat chakra

Sanskrit name	Vishuddha or Vishuddhi
Where is it located?	This chakra is located parallel to your thyroid gland, just near your throat.
Which organs does this chakra govern?	Mouth, gums, teeth, trachea, thyroid, vertebrae, neck, throat, oesophagus, parathyroid and hypothalamus.
How does it influence your body, mind and soul?	Sense of security, independence, self-expression, loyalty, communication, planning and organization
How does an imbalance of this chakra impact you?	Flu, fever, sore throat, swollen glands, thyroid imbalance, laryngitis, scoliosis, mouth ulcers, gum problems, voice problems, tooth problems, faith, criticism, addiction and decision making
Symbol	A circle within a descending triangle

The throat chakra or the fifth chakra is central to your will power and communication. Your struggle to make a choice and execute a decision stems from this energy center. It is also responsible for your faith – in fear and in the Divine power. Your ability to communicate the truth and voice your opinions is dependent on your throat chakra. It also enables you to receive and absorb information. A clear throat chakra allows you to express your truth without any worry of what other people may think or say. In contrast, a blocked throat chakra creates anxiousness about how other people react to your views and this leads you to restrain yourself.

The color 'BLUE' elevates this chakra and water is the prime factor involved in this stimulation. Blue is not a natural color in food, however, tart and tangy fruits such as lemons, limes and grapefruit, salt, lemongrass, fruit juices and herbal tea boost this chakra. Blue colored clothes and gemstones such as sapphire and blue agate enhance the positive effects of this throat chakra. Aromatherapy oils such as chamomile, geranium, peppermint, cypress and mint can also boost the powers of this energy center.

The sixth chakra or the brow chakra

Sanskrit name	Ajna (it is also called the third eye chakra)
Where is it located?	It is located on the forehead, in between your eyes
Which organs does this chakra govern?	Neurological systems, brain, pituitary gland, pineal glands, ear, nose and eyes
How does it influence your body, mind and soul?	Sense of trust, intuition and coordination
How does an imbalance of this chakra impact you?	Discipline, sleep disorders, concept of judgement and reality, emotional intelligence, confusion, blindness, stroke, seizure, brain tumor, arrogance, pride, learning disabilities and sleep disorders
Symbol	Descending triangle within a circle

The sixth chakra or the brow chakra enables you to put things into perspective and is a key to learning and wisdom. This chakra is responsible for your intuitive intelligence and universal consciousness. Your third eye chakra helps you to differentiate between reality and fantasy. It also enables you to evaluate your attitudes and beliefs. When the flow of energy is blocked through this chakra, you experience a sense of distrust and self-doubt. An open and clear chakra enables you to connect with your inner wisdom and guides you in the choices you make.

This chakra is elevated by a deep 'INDIGO' color. Indigo colored clothes and stones like Amethyst, Tourmaline and Tanzanite enliven the third eye chakra. It is also present in foods such as dark grapes, blackberries, blueberries, grape juice, lavender, red wine and poppy seeds. Aromatherapy oils such as tourmaline, tanzanite and amethyst can elevate the powers of this energy center.

The seventh chakra or the crown chakra

Sanskrit name	Sahasrara
Where is it located?	It is located at the top of your head and connects to your central nervous system via the hypothalamus and the thalamus
Which organs does this chakra govern?	Central nervous system, pineal gland, top center of your head, midline above your ears
How does it influence your body, mind and soul?	Integration of your complete self, universal consciousness, physical knowledge and wisdom
How does an imbalance of this chakra impact you?	Chronic exhaustion linked to physical ailments, brain disorders, coordination problems, photo-sensitivity, mental sickness, epilepsy, ethics, lack of purpose.
Symbol	A thousand petaled lotus

The crown chakra is your connection to your spiritual nature which in turn enables spirituality to become an integral portion of your physical life. This chakra brings about a spiritual awakening in your consciousness and connects you to the greater cosmic energy. It facilitates enlightenment and knowledge and helps in diffusing the other six chakras below it. The crown chakra is also known as the 'Thousand Petaled Lotus,' which spurts open when you remember your true nature and experience enlightenment.

The key color of this chakra is 'VIOLET' and then 'WHITE'. These colors enable this chakra to enhance its powers. Violet stones of Diamond or Quartz Crystals and aroma oils such as Lavender, Magnolia and Jasmine can enhance your crown chakra. Wearing colored clothes and using incenses such as myrrh, sage, juniper and frankincense enable the free flow of energy in this Spiritual Communication Center.

Balancing the seven chakras

Do you think it is possible to balance something that you cannot see? Will you be able to open up these chakras without getting a feel of what they look like? More importantly, do you even know if your chakras need healing or opening up? Are they blocked presently?

These are difficult questions with an easy answer. To figure out if your chakras (or energy centers in your body) are blocked, all you need to do is look around yourself. How are you doing in terms of your career and relationships? Are you satisfied with your wealth and health? Can make enough time for fun and spiritual fulfillment both? Overall, are you satisfied with the quality of your life? Or do you see yourself struggling in any area of life?

Okay, you have a great career, but are you able to balance your work and life? Alright, you have lost your job and are aware of your artistic skills. Can you monetize these?

How about taking a few minutes to ponder on your life and satisfaction in general? Even if a little something of this seems 'not so great', it indicates a blocked chakra.

The purpose of chakras or the seven energy wheels spinning from your spine towards your head is to channelize the energy wherever it is required. Each chakra links to a specific area in your body and also connects to your specific life situations.

Have you ever experienced traffic jams? Consider a case of a car that is stuck halfway at the traffic intersection. Can you view the traffic disruptions in all directions? And isn't this chaos is only present at the traffic signal? Cross the signal and everything seems to be ok! That is how chakras function.

One blocked chakra can lead to an imbalance on both the sides. The result of this blockage is an increased level of stagnant energy in certain areas and a diminished level in certain other areas. And this leads to poor health, unwelcome life circumstances and lack of well-being.

The problems occurring in your life can be traced to several blocked chakras or only one of these. Is it possible to eliminate this blockage? Well, you have to clear your chakras or open up your chakras through loads of positive changes that begin within your own self. You may try and move places, acquire a new business, change your job, get a wardrobe makeover or get into a new relationship and yet experience no change in your life. This often leads you wondering about the reason. The answer lies in your chakras. You will need to address the energy imbalance in your body, implying you will need to heal yourself through chakras and try and open up your blocked chakras.

Here are some strategies that can enable you to achieve balance in your life by clearing your chakras or the energy centers:

Energy healing techniques: These include Reiki and acupuncture. Energy healers can help you open up your chakras once they sense any blockage. They deploy specific tools that include crystals, gemstones, fine needles, pressure or touch and intention. Crystals are chosen based on the vibrations of these seven chakras. Pressure, touch or needles work through physically stimulating your meridians. Meridians are specific points that enable you to channel your energy towards the chakras. The most important tool here is intention which would imply concentrated emotions or thoughts.

Through the process of Reiki healing, spirit energy is sent to your body; this in turn concentrates itself in areas that require it the most.

Color therapy: Do you perceive certain colors as soothing, relaxing or energizing? On the other hands, do certain colors irritate you, bore you or make you feel a little off? This is not a result of coincidence and is based on the energy levels within your chakras. Each color possesses an explicit vibrational quality that can be utilized to balance a chakra in a manner that it resonates with the color. Remember, each chakra has a specific color. You could use certain colors in your clothing or the environment in order to provide support to a blocked chakra. How about including colorful fruits and veggies in your diet? They serve dual purpose: nutrition and chakra balancing. Isn't it a win-win situation?

Sound Therapy: Sound therapy works through the power of your intuition and the vibrations that you can feel. Sometimes, you want to listen to really loud, energetic music. And then, there are times when you require some soothing and calm music. Listen to your body, go with your intuition and do what feels right. If possible, try and listen to recorded sounds of chimes, bells, Tibetan singing bowls etc.

Visualization: Visualization is one of the most powerful tools towards balancing your chakras. You should memorize the functions and significance of each chakra and then visualize yourself as someone who has achieved perfection in each area. Your current situation may not be the ideal one and you may be disturbed, guilty, unhappy or tired. Try and align your energy with what you want to achieve – this will be the ideal situation that you should visualize yourself in. Do you want to achieve happiness, success, love, health, wealth and general well-being? Visualize your success, feel each chakra working towards imparting that ultimate energy to your body, mind and soul. Let the power of visualization empower you to achieve greatest happiness through chakra balancing.

Positive affirmations: These are powerful mantras, chants or quotes that encourage you to stimulate positive emotions. You can choose any powerful mantra that you like or even create your own. It just has to be strong enough to provoke positive emotions in your body and mind. You may want to use these affirmations in your meditation or yoga practice. It is a good idea to say them loud to yourself, filled with feelings and focussed on the outcome that you desire. How about a positive affirmative sentence three times a day standing in front of the mirror? Try it in order to experience the magic!

Yoga: Yoga can work as your outside -in approach to balance the chakras by achieving physical and mental balance. It helps you concentrate through balancing your mind and enables you to achieve the perfect mind body synchronization.

Breathing meditation: The simplest known way to achieve calm is through breathing meditation. Focussing on your breath allows you to slow down your heart rate, which in turn empowers your body and mind to slow down. Want to achieve inner peace, healing and tranquillity at a moment's notice? Try deep breathing, it works!

Daily practice of some of these techniques along with some guided discipline is all that is required in order to achieve perfect harmony through chakras.

Chakra mudras

Mudras are specific positions of your hand that instigate a positive flow of energy and are used to balance your seven chakras. The simplest, most impactful and universally acclaimed mudras that can be used independently, during your meditation practice or as a part of any chakra healing strategy are given below:

Pran mudra for the first chakra or the root chakra

This mudra is achieved through touching the tips of the thumb, ring finger and little finger (or pinky finger) together. You can even rest your thumb over the ring finger and pinky finger together.

You should now lengthen your index finger and the middle finger.

Now keep both your hands rested at your sides or your lap, incorporating them into a standing meditation pose or any other pose that is relaxing and comfortable to you.

Practicing deep and mindful breathing meditation at this time can awaken your Pran Mudra's strong grounding impact. This also activates the lesser chakras present in the soles of your feet and enables your life force energy to flow freely through your system. It flushes out any negative energy present in the system and enables you to feel really strong and centered.

Dhyani mudra for the second chakra or the Sacral Chakra

The Dhyani mudra is practiced through placing the back of one on your hand over the palm of the other hand. In this mudra, the tips of the thumbs of both the hands touch each other. Your middle finger, ring finger and little finger can lie on either hand (positioning top of each other). The thumb and index fingers are touched together on either hand in order to form a circle.

It is noticed that during a chakra imbalance, the sacral chakra is normally the first one to be impacted. This mudra strengthens the sacral chakra, creates a sense of responsibility and sharpens concentration. It helps in eliminating any kind of distraction.

Hakini Mudra for the third chakra or the Solar Plexus Chakra

This mudra is practiced by holding both the hands up and allowing the tips of each corresponding finger to touch each other gently.

Your hands can be kept suspended in this position just in front of your abdomen or you can rest them on your lap. Focus on your comfort here and place your hands in the manner they feel most comfortable.

Balancing this chakra helps in transmitting the balance and energy to the chakras above and below this one. Practice of this mudra leads to emotional stability and balance. It also nurtures a feeling of empathy in your body and creates more sensitiveness within you. It also ensures that you stay in control of yourself and are able to exercise control over your emotions.

Gyan Mudra for the fourth chakra or the Heart Chakra

This mudra is practiced by joining the tips of your thumb and index finger on both the hands together. The other three fingers must also be joined and then extended straight up together. Now, let your hands remain in this pose over your heart.

The Gyan Mudra helps to nurture feelings of love and compassion. It enables you to be generous and encourages you to share your happiness with others. This brings in more mindfulness and awareness towards your surroundings. Practicing this mudra enables you to bestow others with the same positive energy that you possess and treat everyone with love and kindness.

Gyan Mudra for the fifth chakra or the Throat Chakra

You can use the Gyan Mudra for healing and balancing your fifth chakra or the throat chakra. The hands pose and the placement of your hands is similar to the manner above.

You understand that the Gyan mudra opens up the path of love, understanding, empathy and compassion. Did you know that practicing Gyan mudra can enhance your communication skills as well? It calms you and supports you in the absorption of any new learnings and knowledge. You get to share your ideas and thoughts in addition to compassion and love.

Shambavi Mudra for the sixth chakra or the Third Eye Chakra

The Shambavi mudra may feel a little unnatural and strange in the beginning, but it is considered as an effective mudra that can be applied during your meditative practice.

It encourages you to roll your eyes upwards, keeping them open. Your focus should be on ensuring that your eyes do not get strained and are yet rolled upwards. This enables your eyes to move their focus from the surrounding and try and see the center of your forehead where your third eye is located. It is a little advanced mudra and needs a little more practice.

Practicing this mudra empowers you to utilize your full potential, increase your intuition and reach a greater level of awareness.

Akasha Mudra and Khechari Mudra for the seventh chakra or the Crown Chakra

In order to practice this mudra you would need to roll your eyes upwards in a similar manner as in Shambavi mudra. Your hand pose should allow you to touch the thumb of your hand to the middle finger of the same hand with the remaining fingers extended outside. You can even touch the thumb of your hand to the ring finger and the middle finger together, leaving the other two fingers extended.

This mudra enables you to balance your spirit energy along with elevating your sensitivity.

Using the Mudras

You can use these mudras as a part of your regular meditation session. You may choose to perform all the mudras starting from the Pran mudra for your root chakra and gradually moving to the Akasha mudra for the crown chakra. You can even dedicate an entire meditation session to one mudra. Mudras also enable you to visualize the location of each chakra along with visualizing the benefits and the color of chakras through the positions of your hand. Encourage yourself to visualize your perfectly balanced chakras. You can even utilize the power of chakra chants and invoke the healing power of sound.

Your intuition can help you decide which chakra needs more care and balancing. It is a good idea to try and attain harmony amongst all seven chakras.

Chakra chants

Balancing and opening the chakras can be achieved through various methods. One prominent way to achieve this harmony is through the use of sound. Chakra chants can be used as a part of your meditation practice and can enable you to achieve balance and harmony in a healing manner.

Before we get into the specifics of chakra chants and how to use them, it is important to understand that the sole thing that can impact chakra balance and healing is your intention. Your intention, in combination with the frequency of your chakra chant, will lead to ultimate healing. Scepticism indicates a less pure intention which results in slower healing. You should focus on using your intention in a powerful manner so that you achieve the desired healing and balance.

What is the best way to set your intentions for healing? Well, try doing it through the positive affirmation. Tell yourself positive things in present tense. Example could include – 'I am healing myself through this chant' or 'I am completely healed of all disease and negativity' or 'I am experiencing a completely balanced life through this chakra chant'. The words that you use and the manner in which you use these words are an important factor in deciding how the healing energy will circulate through your body. Visualizing yourself completely healed and perfectly balanced impacts in a positive manner and enables you to achieve perfect harmony.

The primary focus, therefore, should be on ramping up your positive emotions.

How is sound used for healing?

Everything on this planet is in a constant state of motion and possesses its exclusive frequency that is caused due to movement and transmission of energy.

Can you imagine yourself listening to an orchestra? What do you experience? Do you notice all musical instruments playing in perfect rhythm, each one trying to contribute towards the creation of the miraculous music that you are listening to?

Now imagine your body as an orchestra. Did you know that each organ in your body, every single body system and each cell possesses its own sound, similar to the individual instruments in the orchestra trying to create a perfect rhythm? Can you feel your body 'humming' to the tune of its various organs in the most miraculous manner? It sounds magically harmonious when it is in perfect health.

Now think about one instrument in this orchestra going out of balance. Wouldn't you be able to spot the discorded tune immediately? The same thing happens in your body too. A small symptom such as a feeling of lethargy may cause disharmony in the entire body. And quite often, you dismiss these subtle signs until something major happens. This 'major' thing is what you normally term as a disease – a result of an 'out of tune' body system.

And all it requires is focus that helps in bringing the system back in tune or harmony. This begins with your intention and usage of specific sounds.

Bija Mantras or the seed mantras

Bija mantras are the mantras that are chanted to clear, heal and open your chakras. 'Bija' is the Sanskrit word for the English word 'Seed'. This seed empowers you to implant the most important energy or vital force in your body. It enables each chakra to align itself with the other chakras in order to achieve the desired harmony and balance.

You can choose to chant these Bija Mantras or Seed Mantras individually in order to strengthen a particular chakra or they can be chanted as a series that empowers you to balance your seven chakras. How you want to chant these Bija Mantras is up to you. You may choose to chant these aloud or in your mind, depending on your preference. Want an added dose of energy? Visualize the location, color and positive impact of each chakra as you chant the corresponding Bija mantra.

- In order to chant the Bija Mantra, start at the root chakra and recite the sound LAM. Let this sound be emphatic and short ('m' should not linger).

- Now, move up to your sacral chakra by reciting VAM.

- Next, stimulate your solar plexus chakra through the chant of RAM.

- Move to the heart chakra now using the sound YAM (this is pronounced as 'yum')

- Open your throat chakra by the chant of HAM (this is pronounced as 'hum')

- Now, stimulate your third eye chakra with the sound of OM.

- And finally, open your crown chakra through an extended sound of OM or through complete silence.

Throughout the process, visualize caring, loving energy traveling through your body into the universe. Tell yourself that you can feel this positive energy traveling from your root chakra to your crown chakra and then into the universe.

If you choose to chant these mantras in a series, you can replace the OM or the silence of the crown chakra with "SO HUM" which implies "I am that" – this is used as a positive affirmation that you ARE these chants, you ARE this energy, and that you ARE perfect. Don't forget to visualize yourself in great health as you chant these mantras.

Practicing this chakra chant for a few minutes every day leads to harmony and happiness. You can chant everywhere – in your car, during lunch time, while doing the dishes, while folding your laundry, while baking and cooking, while walking or running, while traveling, as a part of your meditation or yoga practice or even while bathing! Chant these Bija Mantras during peak traffic time and experience the magic these bring into your life – you will feel relaxed and calm in no time! Stressed out at this moment? Try the Bija Mantra chant, it will work wonders and you will notice your stress melt away in seconds.

Treat your body as the most marvelous orchestra and strive hard to maintain the perfect rhythm.

Yoga for chakras

Did you know that one of the greatest and proven methods to boost your chakras is through yoga? The practice of yoga empowers you to balance the elements of air, fire, earth, water, light, sound and thoughts by working its way up your spine. Pranayama, meditation, chanting and asanas are some fantastic yoga tools to help you sail through the chakra system and boost your life force or energy centers.

Out of the various types of yoga, Kundalini yoga is a great method to open up your chakras. It is also termed as the *'yoga of awareness'* and means awakening your Kundalini or inner force, knowledge and consciousness. Kundalini yoga focusses on the flow of the vital life force or the prana from the base of your spine to the crown of your head.

Here are seven yoga poses for stimulating the power of the seven chakras in your body:

Yoga for the root chakra

This chakra is located at the base of your spine and is the force that keeps us grounded to the Earth. It forms the base of your existence. The *Setu Bandha Sarvangasana,* also called *back*bend asana or the Bridge pose requires your feet to be confidently grounded and your spine raised. This opens up your root chakra and focusses energy towards it.

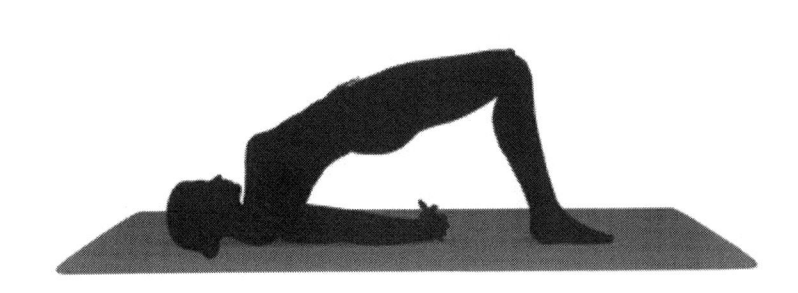

- Lie flat on your back with your hands placed palm down by your sides.
- Now, bend your knees, bringing your feet closer to your bottom. Do ensure that your feet are parallel on the ground.
- Next, press your feet confidently against the ground, lifting your hips up towards the ceiling.
- Now, interweave your fingers under your body, extend your arms and press them down on to the ground, enabling you to elevate your chest and back.
- Move your chest towards your chin, carefully rolling your shoulders.
- Stay in this position and breathe.
- Release the pose, by moving your hands into the palm down position beside you and bringing your upper back, middle back and then the lower back down. Lower your hips too.
- Keep your knees bent before you allow them to touch and rest.

Yoga for the sacral chakra

The second chakra is also known as the sacral chakra and is located in your lower abdomen, near the womb area. It connects you to your inner child. The cobra pose of the Bhujangasana lays stress on the region that helps in opening open up this chakra.

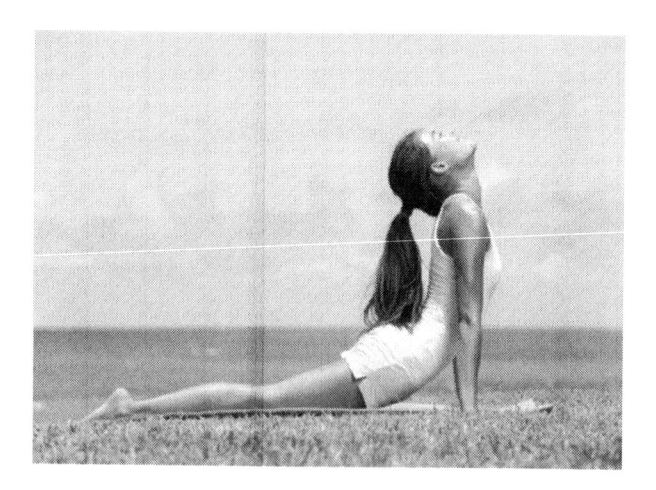

- Lie flat on your stomach with your palms facing down on either side just under your shoulders. Your elbows should touch your body.
- Do not use your hand for support and start lifting your upper body in this order – forehead, nose, chin, shoulders and chest. Lift it as much as possible using the muscles in your back.

- Press your palms down on the floor when you are unable to go higher and use the support of your arms to move your chest higher and forward. Do take care that your elbows are touching your sides and not far from your body.
- Your legs and the pelvic bone should firmly touch the ground and should not be raised.
- Next, open your chest a little further by rolling your shoulders back and looking upwards.
- Breathe normally.
- Use the support of your arms to lower your body and then rest with your hands near your shoulders.

Yoga for the Solar Plexus Chakra

The Solar Plexus Chakra is located in the area near your navel and is responsible for your will power. The bow pose or Dhanurasana is a great way to boost the power of this chakra.

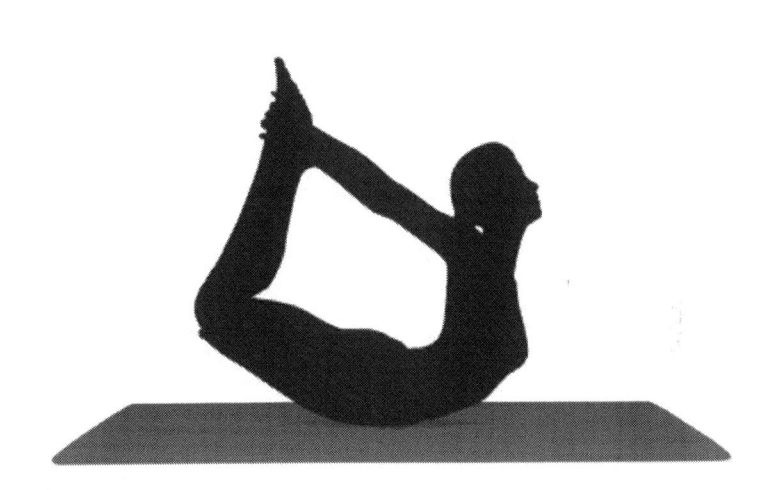

- Lying flat on your stomach, stretch your arms by your sides.
- Stretch your arms back and hold your ankles, breathing normally.
- Lift your legs up from the thighs raise your torso, while inhaling your breath. Do not use your arms in order to pull your legs.
- Open up your chest, lifting your torso further up and breathe deeply, maintaining this pose.
- To release- lower your thighs so that they touch the floor and release your ankles to rest.

Yoga for the heart chakra

The heart chakra is considered as the storehouse of your energy. It is also called the center of empathy, compassion, healing and love and forms a link between your body and spirit. The Ustrasana or the camel pose enables you to elevate your chest towards the sun and is beneficial in opening this chakra.

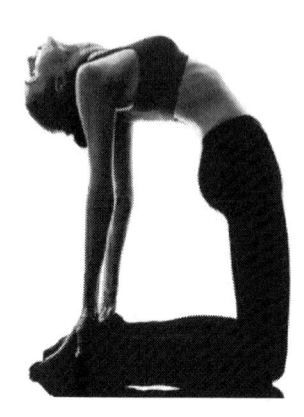

- Begin with a kneeling pose.
- Now move your arms behind you and open up your chest looking up and backwards
- Hold your heels one at a time and keep your hips pushed forward so they are aligned with your knees.
- Move your head back and open your throat, and chest towards the sky.
- Breathe normally.
- To release, raise your head up and release your heels one by one.
- Come back to the original kneeling pose.
- Rest in this pose.

Yoga for the throat chakra

The throat chakra is considered as the center of your communication and includes the neck region along with the throat, thyroid, trachea, vertebrae, neck and mouth. It is also linked to your shoulders, arms, and hands. The fish pose or Matsyasana is therefore a good posture to open up and stimulate this chakra.

- Lie on your back and keep your arms by your sides.
- Now, slowly raise yourself onto your elbows.
- Place your arms under your back as near to your body as possible, and keep your palms under your buttocks, pressing down on the floor. Concentrate your weight on your elbows and lower your body back while elevating your chest.

- Try and look backwards and try dropping the crown of your head onto the floor and opening up your throat.
- Press your forearms further and raise your elbows, opening up your chest a little more.
- To release, gently lower your head and body and come back to a sleeping position.

Yoga for the brow chakra
The third-eye chakra or the brow chakra is located in your forehead, between your eyes and is instrumental towards your learning and wisdom. It enables you to put things into perspective.

- Start by sitting on your heels and keep your back straight.
- Take your hands behind you and interweave your fingers together. Pull your chest up and your arms down in order to elongate your spine further.
- Now roll back and open up your chest, squeezing your shoulder blades together.
- Next bend forward from your hips. Keep your bottom firmly seated with your arms still locked behind you.
- Enable your back to round over your knees and place your forehead (third eye) to the ground.
- Slowly extend your arms up behind you in a manner that your hands reach towards the ceiling with your shoulders still rolled back and arms straight.
- Hold this position and breathe
- To release, slowly bring your body back to the seated position.

Yoga for the crown chakra
The Crown Chakra is your connection to your spiritual self and rules your connection to the central nervous system. The headstand pose called *Salamba Sirsasana* or meditation in half or full lotus position helps stimulate the crown chakra. However, you may want to continue the below mentioned steps in order to stimulate your crown chakra. These steps are in continuation to the steps mentioned above in the asana (pose) for brow chakra.

- Before releasing your arms down from the last pose, elevate your buttocks up from the heels to come onto your knees.
- Roll your head from your forehead and place your arms stretched overhead.
- Now hold this pose and breathe, focussing on the crown of your head.
- To release, bring your body back into the seated position.

The final word

Did you know that you can keep your chakras balanced and open through positivity? You often tell yourself that you are impacted by the negativity in your environment. However, it is never an outside environment that makes you positive or negative. This is because positivity is a state of mind; it is an attitude or the manner in which you choose to live your life. You can either choose to be a positive person or a negative person. There may be days when you would feel sad and negative, however, that does not imply that you are a negative person. On the other hand, your feeling happy on a certain day does not make you a positive person overall.

Consciously choosing to keep a positive attitude creates a positive life experience. Here are some proven strategies to elevate that element of positivity in your life:

- **Repositioning your thoughts:** Whenever your thoughts lead you to frustration, anger, or grief, try and reposition them to doing something totally unrelated. Consciously choose not to think about the situation causing anger or grief.

- **Focus on positive outcome for negative thoughts too:** Yes! This may sound a little weird but each thought that comes into your mind is linked to an outcome. Negative thoughts have an outcome too. Consciously think about positive outcomes for negative thoughts too. Tell yourself – whatever the thought, the result has to be positive and that is all that matters.

- **Utilize the power of positive affirmations and visualization:** Visualize your chakras in harmony and balance with each other. Focus on positive affirmations. Always tell yourself how good things are at the moment and visualize how they can be better.

- **Count your blessings:** Practice gratitude. There are a thousand reasons you can be grateful for. Think about the positive things in your life, the relationships that you value and the material things that you possess and be grateful for everything. Let positivity fill your body, mind and soul.

Always remember that your thoughts and emotions can impact your chakras. Is it then not a great idea to let positive thoughts impact your chakras in a positive manner and help in creating the sense of balance and harmony within your chakras?

A Preview to Coconut Oil

12. Because of coconut oil's moisturizing properties, it can be used to soothe skin conditions such as eczema and psoriasis. Eczema is a blanket term for conditions that cause inflammation and irritation of the skin. Atopic Dermatitis is the most common type and it is seen mostly in people who have inherited allergies such as asthma or hay fever. The disease can be controlled and most babies who have the disease outgrows it by the age of 10. Some adults have to deal with it the rest of their life. The skin can appear thick, dry, and scaly. Dark skin can cause the area to become lighter or darker, and in people with fair skin the area can become red or brown. The itchy rash appears in infants scalps and face causing crusty, runny patches. Coconut oil is a natural treatment for eczema. The oil will stop the flaking and itch of eczema. Massage it deep into the effected area. Apply it at least 4 times a day and at bedtime. Keep the area moist by applying a bandage. You will have to make sure that you see your doctor regarding the cause of your eczema and avoid the allergic causes. They could be certain materials, perfumes, or foods. Psoriasis is a skin disorder that is persistent and hard to be treated. When you have psoriasis your skin cells grow 10 times faster than they usually do causing the cells to die when they reach the surface of the skin. The skin then becomes raised and red sometimes cracking open, becoming scaly, painful and irritated. The patches can cover larger parts of the body when they merge together. Other symptoms include discoloration of fingernails and toenails, and scaly, crusty patches on the scalp. The cause of psoriasis has been hard to pinpoint. Some believe that it is associated with psoriatic arthritis that causes painful, swelled joints. The condition comes and goes and it is frustrating when someone is trying to treat the condition. Psoriasis can be caused by streptococcal infection, emotional stress, or even problems with the immune system. Psoriasis tends to be genetic such as dermatitis. Again, the essential fatty acids in coconut oil help boost the immune system. It also can be used topically on the skin as a treatment. Consume the oil as well. It is recommend that 3 tablespoons of extra virgin coconut oil should be taken per day. Use topically after a shower or bath. The patches will begin to dry up, and, in the mean time, they will be softer and less irritated.

13. Arthritis is the leading cause of disability in the United States today. Finding a good anti-inflammatory for arthritis these days can be hard to

do. Drug companies have been in the news recently for putting medicines on the market that aren't safe and cause other health problems. Arthritis is a joint disorder that causes pain and inflammation in one or all of the joints in your body. There are different types of arthritis such as Rheumatoid arthritis, Osteoarthritis, and genetic types of arthritis that causes the disease to attack the joints of children and adults alike. Damage can also be done to your cartilage causing stiffness as well. The damage and stiffness can cause you to have problems handling basic daily chores such as brushing your teeth, typing, and walking. As we have discussed, coconut oil is an anti-inflammatory. You can use coconut oil along with aloe Vera to reduce inflammation in the joints. Simply massage into the effected area. It also strengthens bones and can help soothe sore, stiff joints. Use coconut oil with camphor as a pain relieving agent. Massage the mixture on the joints that are effected. The camphor will help increase blood supply and the warmth of the coconut oil will relieve the pain. Coconut oil can be used after a bath or shower to help with stiff joints. It also increases circulation and can be used before exercise. Mix a bit of essential oil in and it smells much more pleasant than some store bought arthritis medications.

14. Hemorrhoids are common and you can use natural coconut oil to relive the discomfort. Hemorrhoids can be internal or external and are caused by a variety of reasons including pregnancy, heredity, and chronic diarrhea or constipation. They are very painful, and can become so bad that surgery may become an option for relief. A hemorrhoid is caused by too much pressure being placed on the rectum. Tissues inside the rectum will fill with blood to help with bowl movements, however, when pressure is placed on them, they swell and stretch causing pain. They can be identified by itching, pain in the rectal area, and bleeding while having a bowl movement. Blood will appear on the toilet paper if that happens. Coconut oil can relieve the inflammation when used topically. You can put the oil on a cotton ball and place it against the hemorrhoid 2 or 3 times a day. This should give relief from itching and inflammation.

15. When your little one has an ear infection it hurts you to watch him hurt. Coconut oil can be a very good natural remedy for an ear infection. Because coconut oil is anti-bacterial, anti-fungal, anti-parasitic, antimicrobial, and anti-protozoa, it kills just about everything. Some parents may be concerned with the over use of antibiotics and the risk that they cause for candida overgrowth and other side effects. Warm the oil until it becomes a liquid. Make sure it isn't too warm.

Draw the oil into an eye dropper or syringe and put a few drops into the ear. Make sure they are lying comfortably and let them stay there until the oil is absorbed into the ear. Put a bit of a cotton ball in the ear to keep the oil from running out. If for any reason you believe that the eardrum is ruptured, or if the earache is accompanied by a high fever, check with your healthcare provider immediately.

If you enjoyed this preview click the link below to get this best selling book:

Coconut Oil - 101 Miraculous Coconut Oil Benefits, Cures, Uses, and Remedies

Thank YOU!

Thank you for checking out this book. I pour my heart into all my work.

IF you enjoyed this book please take a few seconds to leave a quick review.

To your health,

Victoria Lane

Made in the USA
Lexington, KY
23 June 2018